Crossing the Minefield

One Widow's Journey

Melinda Richarz Lyons

Crossing the Minefield
One Widow's Journey

ISBN: 978-1-61752-130-0
TreasureLine Publishing
www.TreasureLinePublishing.com

www.MelindaLyons.com
www.TreasureLineBooks.com

Cover Design: Laura J. Miller, www.AnAuthorsArt.com
Interior Formatting: Ellen C. Maze, www.ellencmaze.com

The views expressed in this work are solely those of the author

PRINTED IN THE UNITED STATES OF AMERICA

To Sidney Johnson Bailey

What other widows are saying about

Crossing the Minefield

Your book was so on target. You have no idea what it meant to me to read through my tears of someone else's journey that so closely parallels mine.

I had a good cathartic cry over your book—read and clung to every single word. Your words have given me hope.

Thank you from the bottom of my shattered heart for caring enough to help me through this hateful journey. I know that I will survive this.

This is SO my story and I can relate. You've made a difference in my life.

Chapter List

1

This Can't Be Happening

When I woke up that late November day, I realized my husband Sid, an early-riser, was still in bed. *Maybe he is just tired*, I thought. He had been so busy with his business lately. So I got up and went down to make the coffee. It was just a typical fall morning in Murfreesboro, Tennessee—chilly and damp. And it was still dark outside.

I walked back upstairs and said something like, "Hey, are you awake?" I turned on the bedroom light. Sid didn't respond and so I touched him. He didn't move. Not at all. I remember the total stillness in his body.

After that everything was a complete blur. Somehow I managed to dial 911. I remember the operator asking me if there was someone else in the house to help me. I know she asked about a neighbor, but I don't recall if I gave her Marsha's number or not. I am sure the operator told me to try to roll him over, but I couldn't. He outweighed me by a good one hundred pounds.

I was alone. I was screaming. I was begging. I was crying. I know that. The next thing I knew, my neighbor Marsha was at my door in her pajamas yelling, "What's wrong?" The operator had called her.

We struggled to get Sid turned over and then frantically tried to give him CPR with the operator's instructions. But it was obvious when we rolled him over that he was gone. I kept pleading with God not to take him, but I knew it was too late.

The paramedics came, and as they carried Sid down the stairs, I fell to my knees and prayed. *God, please give me a miracle.* They loaded him into the ambulance and told us to get ready to go to the hospital. I threw clothes on over my pajamas. Marsha was gone—following us in her car, while I rode in the front of the ambulance.

It seemed like it took forever to get to the hospital. *What was taking so long? Why didn't people get out of the way? God, please don't take him. Please!* I kept silently begging.

When they pulled him out of the ambulance at the emergency room entrance, I saw his arm flop off the gurney. So lifeless. We went to the waiting room and prayed and cried and begged some more.

The night before flashed through my mind. It had been so ordinary. We watched *Antiques Roadshow,* and Sid teased and played with our little cat, Helen, like he did every night. I don't know what we talked about. I wish I could remember. *Did we say "I love you"? I doubt it. Who says that on an ordinary night while you are doing ordinary things? God, I wish I could remember.*

I wanted to keep thinking about the night before so I shut my eyes. Maybe if I kept them shut, this would all go away. *Please God, make him alive again like he was last night.* I held onto Marsha as tightly as I could and we waited and waited. It was agonizing.

After what seemed like an eternity, the room was suddenly full of people wearing scrubs. They didn't have to tell me that my prayer for a miracle was not answered. I could see it in their eyes. I think I shouted, "God, no!"

"All our efforts to save him failed." The words echoed in my head. The doctor said Sid never got a pulse back. He asked a lot of questions. "Had he been ill? Had he complained? Did he have a history of heart disease?"

"No! No! No!" I screamed. "He had a stress test two months ago for God's sake! He did just fine on that!"

The doctor explained that Sid probably had a massive heart attack. He most likely died in his sleep. The blessing was that he probably felt no pain and didn't know what happened. The paramedics were still there. One—a woman, sat next to me and held me. A nurse was there, I think, and asked if she could get me anything. *Yes, you fool. Bring me my husband.* I remember Marsha saying it just wasn't right. I had lost my dad just six weeks earlier. *How could Sid be dead, too?* We had no children. We had been married almost thirty-eight years. I cried, "He is all I have!" *How could he be gone at fifty-six? Just like that? No warning. God, how could you do this to me*?

Marsha's minister arrived and they knelt down in front of me, praying out loud. Marsha's words came out in sobs. I remember how they tried to hold my legs down because they were jerking so violently I was literally falling off the chair.

They asked if I wanted to see Sid. I did want to say goodbye. I stumbled down a long hall into the darkened room where they had him. He was covered up to his neck, and the tube was still in his mouth. *My poor, sweet baby.*

I remember seeing one little curl sticking up. I thought about how much he hated his curly hair and how he always tried to make it stay down. *He wouldn't like that curl sticking up like that*. But he looked so precious with that little curl over his forehead. I kissed him on the cheek and told him that I loved him. The nurse asked if I wanted to stay with him a while. I said, "No." I didn't want to remember him like that. And then she told me how brave I was. "Brave?" I think I replied. "I don't even know what is going on. This isn't real. This can't be happening!"

2

Close Enough to Perfect for Me

"When I go, don't make me a damn saint!" Sid would sometimes proclaim. It used to irritate him when a widow would suddenly decide that her husband had been the perfect man.

I didn't want to remember Sid lying there lifeless in that tiny, sterile room at the hospital, stripped of his dignity. Instead, I wanted to always remember the strong, confident, proud man he was—imperfections included.

One of the things that had attracted me to Sid in the first place was his confidence. He was only seventeen when we met, yet he had such self assurance. I had none, so that fascinated me. He wasn't cocky—just totally comfortable with who he was. And he took such pride in all aspects of his life from his appearance and how he conducted himself, to his accomplishments. He was everything I wanted to be.

He was also very softhearted. One time he had gone out for a drink with some friends after work. He saw some men throwing something back and forth and went over to investigate. To his horror they were tossing a baby squirrel like a ball, laughing about how the dumb little thing shouldn't have fallen out of his tree.

Sid apparently asked if they would throw the squirrel his way. He grabbed it and headed out of the bar. He met me at our door with a tiny, frightened squirrel in his front pocket. We bottle-fed it for several weeks and then gave the squirrel to some friends who lived in the country. Years later he still talked about that incident. Sid could never come to grips with the fact that people could actually be cruel to animals—or to children and older people for that matter.

I recall another time an old man was trying to cross a street in front of us. A car load of teenagers came roaring up and honked and yelled at the old man as he struggled to get across the road. Sid was furious and called them insensitive, idiotic "low lives."

Sid was the kind of guy who would always be there for you, no matter what. I remember a cousin called him once at about four in the morning in trouble. Sid didn't ask questions—he just jumped in his car and went to her aide. He was strong enough to lean on anytime. I think that is what people loved about him—that combination of softness and strength.

I thought our friend Jeff put it well when he spoke at Sid's memorial. He said "The first time I saw Sid he was walking up to the house, and I was thinking that I didn't want to make that great big, mean-looking guy mad. But after talking with him for about five minutes I realized that Sid did not have a mean bone in his body. He truly was a gentle giant."

Sid's frugal nature was another thing that made him unique. Once when Sid opened his wallet in front of our nephews, they all kidded him by yelling, "Look, moths!" His tight hold on money often got on my nerves, as I had to fight to get him to spend a dime. When my twenty-five-year-old oven stopped working, he had to be convinced that a new one was a necessary expense.

A few months before he died, the muffler fell off his car. Sid threw it in the trunk, because, after all, it would cost a little money to replace it. You could hear him coming from a mile away and it didn't seem to concern him that he might get a ticket. He died with that muffler still in his trunk. It was so typically Sid.

But his determination to hang onto money helped me tremendously when he died. I didn't have a lot of debts, because Sid didn't believe in debts. And I had some money in the bank.

In my eyes, Sid's best quality had to be the fact that he would do things just to make people happy. He didn't have to get anything out of it himself. His only motivation was seeing someone's big beaming smile.

He had a 1965 Impala that was his pride and joy. He had worked many summers to buy it and had fixed it up with all the bells and whistles. It was a totally cool car. That yellow Impala was a source of so many memories. It had black interior and bucket seats. When we were dating, we used to try to ride together in one bucket seat!

My best memory concerning that car was my first birthday after we were married. We were broke, so I didn't expect a gift. Sid had fancy hubcaps on the old Chevy and sold them to buy me a birthday gift. I know what it took for him to part with those hubcaps. But more important to him was the fact that he was coming home with a special gift—a little daisy clock that I still treasure.

Sid was almost too honest. If I asked him "Does my butt look too big in this outfit?" he would say, "Yes, actually it does look pretty big." But then because of his great sense of humor and kind nature, he would add, "But I LOVE your big butt!"

No, Sid wasn't perfect. He could be moody and was very shy. He enjoyed being by himself and had difficulty sometimes interacting with people he didn't know very well. I often had to be social enough for both of us. He snored too loudly, was particular about certain kinds of foods and would throw his dirty clothes on the floor. But his imperfections were minor to me.

It would take me a while to erase that awful picture in my head of someone once so full of life lying dead in the emergency room. Eventually I would be able to recall his beautiful smile and all the wonderful qualities that made Sid close enough to perfect for me. In the meantime, I would have to work through the numbness and shock that followed his untimely death.

3

Everybody's Talking at Me

I remember the sea of faces that seemed to drift past me as I sat at my kitchen table. People touching me, crying, and saying things like, "I'm so sorry. Please let me know what I can do."

I vaguely recall the trip to the funeral home. Thank God for friends. It was two days before Thanksgiving and the closest family member was hundreds of miles away. So I relied on my friends Marsha and Donna to help me make the decisions. What day did I want the funeral? What time? What was Sid's Social Security number? How much education did he have? *What? Who cares?* Oh---for the death certificate.

There were answers to give the funeral director for the obituary. Oh, and would he be cremated? Buried? Where? The questions became echoes that pounded in my head, and I just wanted to lie down somewhere and go to sleep. Maybe when I woke up, this would all just be a bad dream.

I remember people saying that you go through a shock stage after a death—particularly a sudden death. It was more like a nightmare, and it all seemed very surreal. I felt like I was having an out-of-body experience. It was like I was watching some other woman dealing with her husband's premature death.

I know I insisted on talking to family members myself. I remember Marsha calling my brother in Seattle and telling him that Sid had "passed." Then she handed me the phone, and I sobbed and told him to please come as fast as he could.

The phone rang off the wall, and people and food just kept coming. The support and love I got was amazing. Too bad I was in such a daze I didn't really appreciate it at the time.

I look back and I am deeply grateful for the way everyone went "above and beyond" for me. I can't imagine what it would have been like to deal with such a loss without all that help. Neighbors I barely knew brought me casseroles and kind words. Friends scurried around, cleaning and preparing the bedrooms for family members. My co-workers came with food and other items they had purchased after collecting money from everyone. They even thought to purchase paper products to make things easier for us.

When my sister from California arrived, Marsha's son, Bryson, escorted her around town, helping her run necessary errands. That way I could sit at the house and continue to greet the throngs of people who wanted to pay their respects and offer help. I know I probably looked like a zombie, mumbling a response here and there. Later on, people told me about conversations that I had with them. But I don't remember even talking, let alone what I said to anyone. It was like I had taken some kind of mind-altering drug. I couldn't connect with anything or anyone for days.

Everyone was in shock, though. Not to the degree that I was, of course, but disbelief was the reaction of each person who heard the news. Sid was just three weeks away from turning fifty-seven. He was a huge, jolly guy who had played professional football in his younger days. He appeared to be the picture of health. I kept hearing voices asking, "How could he be dead? Can you believe it?"

Shock and disbelief surrounded me the days right after Sid died. I was totally numb. Just like the song said, everybody was talking at me, but I didn't hear a word they were saying.

4

Crossing the Minefield

Most of the literature I read after I lost my husband described the grief process as a roller coaster ride. One day you would think you were making it okay—slowly moving up to a place where you would feel good again. Then suddenly you would go careening down into that deep dark place where you were totally out of control. It wasn't unusual, I discovered, to believe the tiny bit of progress you had made up to that point was gone forever. I felt that way in the months after the shock of Sid's death was just beginning to wear off, but I would describe my emotions a little differently. I think what I went through was what it must be like to try to cross a minefield.

To me, it was more than just experiencing those intense highs and lows. It was the fact that being knocked back down into that awful hole of grief often came from stepping into a situation that took me by surprise and ripped me apart. On the surface, everything looked okay. But I knew the triggers for my grief were all around me—hiding and just waiting to explode like bombs. I would try so hard to be careful and do everything I could to avoid the emotional meltdowns because they were so painful.

Some days, I would just be walking along, believing that I was finally at least trying to get a handle on those terrible emotions. And then boom! I would step right onto one of those triggers, and the bomb would explode in my face—knocking me backwards. I would find myself again on the ground, feeling dismembered, disoriented, and depressed beyond belief.

I tried to be prepared for the obvious

mines. There were certain things I knew would trigger those bombs of emotion, like the first Christmas or birthday without him. But I wasn't prepared at all for some of the mines, because they turned out to be bombshells.

One day I went to Sid's favorite store. No big deal. I was just going to pick up a few groceries. When I entered the store, I smelled the bakery and thought about the little chocolate cupcake he brought me one year for my birthday. I heard the voice of the big guy behind the meat counter—the one who always liked to talk to Sid about football.

Suddenly, I began to sob. I thought I was in a safe area, but that damn mine wasn't where it was supposed to be, and I stepped on it. The grief exploded in my face when and where I wasn't expecting it.

Then there were those moments when I would actually forget what happened. Like one day I was driving home, thinking about something that occurred at work. *Oh, I will have to tell Sid about that.* I pulled into the driveway and realized he was not there and I would never again be able to run in the house and say, "Hey, guess what?" God, those moments caused such horrendous damage.

The minefield could really fool you, too, as time passed. About eight months into my grief, I thought I was on safer ground because I felt like a lot of the most damaging grief bombs had already exploded. But I was wrong. Although the meltdowns at that point were less intense and fewer and farther apart, they still happened. And when they did, I would be caught totally off guard--just like I had been months before at the grocery store.

Two days before the eight-month anniversary of Sid's death, I opened his closet to get the iron. I had done that numerous times before, and I thought I was dealing with seeing his things pretty well. I had not done anything with his clothes, and it seemed to bother me less and less to see them hanging there.

But that day when I opened the closet door, I found myself grabbing the sleeve of his old blue shirt. I rubbed it against my face and smelled it. Even clean, it smelled like Sid. I wrapped the arms of the shirt around me and cried until I couldn't cry anymore. I fell onto the floor, curling up like a baby and feeling that horrible deep hurt again.

Where did that mine come from? I thought I had stepped on all the mines involving his clothes and they were gone. I had been going into that closet for months. I would see his jeans and shirts hanging there and not get upset. *So what happened that time?* I stepped on a mine I didn't see and was blown apart.

Through all my stages of grief, I found that crossing the minefield never ended—it just got easier. I discovered that there would always be mines hiding in places I did not expect. And I would step on one every once in a while.

The minefield would be with me forever. But on my journey, I would learn how to maneuver my way through it and survive.

5

Where Have All the Flowers Gone?

The stages of grief are unique for everyone, and each person goes through them differently. I learned that some people never even go through certain stages, and the order also varies with each individual. Some overlap and you can revisit an earlier stage at any time.

After the shock wore off for me, the worst stage of all set in—depression. I felt all of the things described by the grief experts—emotional pain, hopelessness, anguish, loneliness, despair and discomfort.

I found that the discomfort included physical pain, too. You hurt so much emotionally that it often leads to things like headaches and stomach aches. I couldn't eat, and I rarely slept peacefully for a long time after Sid died.

Sometimes very well-meaning friends would cause me more pain. I learned a lot about what not to say to someone in so much pain. I couldn't stand it when someone would say, "Oh, one of these days you will see a reason for this," or "This is God's plan."

God's plan? Well, then he didn't think much of me, did he? He destroyed my family. Since we had no children, Sid was all I had. To people with children, I would think that losing a child would be the worst thing that could happen to them. For me, it was losing Sid.

When I told my wonderful grief counselor that it upset me deeply when people would say I should have faith and trust in God's plan, she said, "Well, just tell them if this is God's plan, then it sucks!" That may sound offensive to some people, but to me it was exactly what I needed to hear.

For me, it didn't have anything to do with faith or my belief and trust in God. At that point, I did not want to hear that God's plan included hurting me so deeply and turning my life completely upside down and inside out.

But it was almost worse when people stopped saying anything. At first you are surrounded by people who provide love and support. Life goes on as it should. So the visits got fewer and the phone calls less frequent. As all the beautiful flowers I had received began to die, the depression became unbearable.

The house seemed so big and lonely without Sid. I even started missing the fact that he never wiped his feet before he came into the house and threw his big shoes in the middle of the floor. Sometimes I would call his name just to hear the sound of it again.

Sid's brother had died four years before at age fifty. My sister-in-law Becky said that for almost a year she was "completely consumed by sadness." I thought I understood what she meant, but of course at the time, I did not.

I never knew I could hurt that much. Like most people, I had been through some rough times in my life and many family deaths. But the pain of Sid's death was like no other I had ever experienced. I wanted to die. I lost interest in everything. I could not see any hope for the future. I felt isolated and alone, like I was on an island all by myself—suffering like no one else had ever suffered.

I would immediately turn the TV channel if I saw a couple kissing. When two people in public were laughing and holding hands, I wanted to scream, "Stop it! Don't you know my whole world is gone?" I couldn't watch. I no longer had that and it hurt so much. Whenever I heard "Bridge Over Troubled Water"—the song we had played at Sid's memorial, I wanted to call the radio station. I felt like saying, "Don't ever play that song again! Don't you realize that it tears me to pieces when I hear it?"

As the months went by, I also discovered that some of our couple friends drifted away. It was only natural. I wasn't part of a couple anymore. That was a double hurt. And it seemed like people stopped wanting to talk about him. I wanted to talk about Sid all the time then. Maybe it was my way of trying to keep him alive. So it was painful to have to sit and listen to small talk about soccer games and dances.

I tried so hard every day to find a reason to go on. I would wake up in the morning, look up and imagine that Sid was looking down at me. I would pretend that he was telling me, "Get your butt out of bed! I don't want you to lie around and feel sorry for yourself!"

Of course, some days I could not help but feel sorry for myself. Once in a while, I had to stay in bed with the covers over my head. But the more I tried to recover, the better things got. The old saying about time being a great healer is true. I slowly—very slowly--began to inch along and feel like life was worth living again.

Eventually, I learned to accept help and started lifting myself out of the "it's all about me" mode. I even began trying to help other people a little. When those things happened, the island I was on started drifting back to the shore. But it would take a lot to get there, and it all started with my grief group.

6

No One is an Island

I always thought I was the type of person who could probably make it on my own. But on top of the grief over Sid's death, I was struggling with a lot of issues, including the fact that I had never been single.

I had gone from daddy to dormitory to husband. I didn't have a clue how to take care of myself. I would panic over every little thing from balancing the checkbook to fixing a leaky toilet. Sid always did those things. I was the one who kept him fed, did most of the household chores, and bought every gift we ever gave anybody.

Of course it was more complicated than that, but when he was alive, our roles were clear and it was so much easier. Now I had to take on his role, too. I felt overwhelmed and terrified.

Once I stopped being stubborn and got over the idea that I had to "go it alone," things improved. Get the neighbor to show you how to fix the toilet. Ask your brother for help concerning insurance issues. Let you girlfriend take care of your cats so you can take a trip. That is what friends and family are for, I was told over and over. So I started to listen.

One of the best ways I got help was through a local hospice program. Even though Sid had not died from an extended illness, our local hospice offered grief counseling. My friend, Diana, worked for Alive Hospice in a nearby town, and she was the one who put me in touch with Pam.

I had to let go of the perception that it was a "weakness" to ask for help or go for counseling. From the very first session, I found that a professional grief counselor can help you tremendously. Pam was compassionate but realistic. She gave me valuable tools to work with so I could start the healing process. And she let me cry. One day she told me that she would be starting a grief group soon. *A grief group? Now wouldn't that be sort of a pity party thing?* I decided to try it, and that is when my broken heart really began to gradually heal.

At the first session we all sat there in silence and sobbed. Then one person spoke up. I don't even know what was said. All I know is that suddenly I knew I was not alone on this terrible journey. I wasn't crazy, either. Other people had the same feelings I did.

With the help of Pam and another facilitator, Karen, we all discovered that although our paths were different, we had shared emotions and concerns. They in turn validated our feelings and gave us hope and help to go on.

We all had to find our own way to get through this. But we could help each other. And we did. We could confess things and no one would tell. We talked about such personal things, and almost every person in our group admitted thinking about suicide. That was normal, too. When someone you love so deeply dies, you want to die too.

Another important thing that I took to heart from those sessions was the description of the new normal. It had to be a goal for each of us. Plan A was gone. Plan B had to be implemented. Life would never be the same. We were stuck with that fact, and we had no choice in the matter.

As newlyweds, we had all joyfully accepted a new normal way of life as we went from being single to becoming a couple. Now, we had to start all over again and this time it was devastating. This new unwanted life affected everything. Suddenly we had to deal with small changes like the way we bought groceries and cooked, to overwhelming changes like how we would pay our bills.

We each had to find a new way to live. For one person, it might be a new job. For another, it might be a move. Should you wait a year to make a major decision? Not necessarily. It depended on the person. There were no rules. Two members of our group married each other and started a new life together.

Even though each person had a different fork in the road to follow, we were close by. So when one person fell on her road or stepped on one of those damn mines, another would be there quickly to pick her up and help nurse the wounds. We depended on each other as we had never depended on anyone ever before.

7

Lean on Me

The group became a family and long after our official eight week session was over, we continued to meet weekly for dinner. I gave each member a copy of a poem I wrote one night.

Sometimes special people enter our lives
Not by birth or family ties.
They come to us by circumstance
But I don't believe it is just by chance.
I was so consumed with deep despair
When I felt the touch of those who care.
In my darkest hour—so left behind

I was facing a mountain I could not climb.
You reached out to me and I held on tight
And I began to see the light.
I believe my angel up above
Had a hand in all this love.
Through all these tears and tragedy
I found a new meaning for family.

We may not have been bonded by birth or ties, but we were drawn together by our awful similar circumstances. I discovered just how powerful that bond could be. We instinctively held onto each other tightly. Slowly we gained the strength to climb up together out of that seemingly bottomless cavern of grief into the warmth of the new normal light.

There were ten of us—eight women and two men. Most were widows, but one had lost her mother and another had lost her son. I can still see the tears, hear the stories, and recall the joyful memories we shared. It makes me warm with comfort when I think about my support group family.

At one meeting we were asked to bring a photo and share a memory about our loved one. I remember how I enjoyed hearing about so many good times and getting to know each of our members through warm memories.

One group member had been deeply in love with her husband years earlier but they had been torn apart by family members who would not allow them to marry. Later after both had been married and divorced, they found each other again, and did become man and wife. I wept with her as she cried over the years they had lost and smiled with her as she expressed gratitude for the time they eventually shared.

Another woman broke our hearts as she sobbed over the loss of her boyfriend. He had gone back to using drugs and died of an overdose. She felt so guilty about not being able to save him. We all rallied around her and assured her that no one could have prevented his death. I think once she felt our compassion and understanding, she began to forgive herself.

Around Valentine's Day, one of our male members brought us each a lovely poem he had printed off the internet entitled *I'm*

There Inside Your Heart. I framed it next to one of my favorite photographs of Sid.

We had our lighter moments too. One night we were asked to share the first memory we had of our loved one. As we went around the table, most people related a sweet recollection, like "Oh, the first time I saw him, I noticed his wonderful smile." Or, "I instantly felt her kindness."

When it was his turn to speak, our only other male member began to tell about how he was working in a defense plant during the war and saw his future wife on the next line. Thinking he was going to tell something sentimental as the other members had, our facilitator asked, "And what was it about her that you noticed first?"

"Oh," he replied, obviously without thinking. "She had on the tightest sweater I had ever seen!" Of course we all started laughing hysterically as he turned a very deep shade of red. And we never stopped kidding him about his enthusiastic response.

Through each other's eyes we grew to know something about every single person we had lost. We learned about their wonderful qualities and sometimes the ones that were not so wonderful. We found that expressing empathy and leaning on each other were equally great therapy for all of us.

We uncovered our strengths and weaknesses, too. We talked through frustrations and fears, discovering so much about ourselves and how we could—and would--eventually make it through our grief.

United we stand—divided we fall. We lived by those words. We helped each other and in turn helped ourselves. I would discover the healing properties of giving back later on a much more individual basis. But as a group we started by crossing the minefield arm in arm.

About six months into our weekly dinner meetings, we all ended up laughing so hard one night. I don't remember what triggered it, but it felt good. The server came up to our large party and said, "What kind of group is this, anyway?"

"A grief group," someone answered. As the server's jaw dropped, another person asked, "Hey does this mean we are actually starting to see a little bit of the new normal?"

Thank God for the grief support group.

8

Why? Why? Why?

Another thing the grief group and counseling helped me deal with was guilt. I had these awful feelings and questions. *Why couldn't I stop him from dying? Couldn't I see that Sid had a problem? Why didn't I make him quit smoking? Why didn't I make him lose weight?*

For a long time, I felt so much guilt—as if it was my fault that he died. I remember thinking that I should have done something. Maybe there were some things that I could have done differently but it was too late for that.

Looking back, I think there were signs that Sid had heart disease. He did pass his stress test but was told to start living a healthier lifestyle. I remember when he got back from taking the stress test, I asked about it.

Sid said there were many questions, like "Did he have a family history of heart disease?" His answer was, "No." I remember saying, "Are you kidding? Your dad died from a sudden heart attack and so did your grandfather." But it didn't occur to me to make him call the doctor back and insist on further testing. I felt like everyone else did—Sid appeared to be a big, healthy guy, so I really wasn't worried.

Another member of our grief group had lost her son to a sudden heart attack. As we talked about our shared experience, we discovered that both her son and Sid had been unusually cold in the months prior to their deaths. *Was that poor circulation? Did that have something to do with their hearts?* They both seemed to be tired a lot, too. Sid's business had increased tremendously, and I just assumed it was because he was working so hard. The other man's exhaustion also had been attributed to the fact that his work schedule had been so demanding. Both were life-long smokers and didn't exercise. Lots of people sit at a computer all day and smoke. That doesn't mean they are all going to die too young. But our loved ones did. We both thought the same thing. *We should have done something to save them.*

For months after Sid died, I would beat myself up about why I didn't do more. *I was his wife, and I was supposed to protect him! Why didn't I?*

I visited his doctor and took a chance that he would forget about all the patient confidentiality crap and tell me the truth. Had Sid tried to protect me and had he lied about the stress test results? I was relieved that the doctor was willing to talk to me about Sid. Yes, he had warned him about smoking and had put him on medication for high cholesterol. I knew Sid had been taking that faithfully.

Sid had told me the truth. He had passed the stress test. The doctor made me feel better when he admitted that even he did not expect Sid to die from a sudden heart attack at fifty-six. That was when the guilt started to lift. If the doctor couldn't save him, then I was powerless, too.

Again, with the help of counseling and the support I found in others, I slowly started to realize that I could not have changed what happened. If his doctor didn't see red flags, then why would I have been able to?

Sid was a big boy, too. I couldn't make him stop smoking, exercise and lose weight. I had tried. The nagging did no good.

I found myself moving from being consumed by guilt to the anger stage.

9

Damn Him - Damn God - Damn Everybody

Anger seemed to take over my life for a while. I was so mad at Sid for leaving me like that. *How could you do this to me? How could you just go away after being part of my life every single day for almost forty years?*

My guilt turned into rage. *Why didn't you take better care of yourself, Sid? Didn't you care enough about me to stay around? Why didn't you just put those damn cigarettes down? Couldn't you see they were killing you? You could have exercised*! I felt hate in my heart.

One time when I was driving along feeling particularly horrible, I began to scream at him at the top of my lungs. I called him every name in the book and told him how very much I hated him for ruining my life. *We were happy together! How could you just die on me and screw everything up like that?*

I found out later that doing that is what you need to do to make it through the anger stage of the grief process. Yell. Scream. Curse. Grab a pillow and pretend that it is your loved one and start beating the hell out of it. It is okay. Let it out. You have a right to be angry.

I felt guilty about it, but I was also very angry with God. Sid and I were not able to have children, and it took me years to get over my anger about that. I always wanted children, and for a while felt God had denied me happiness. But I had come to accept the fact that Sid and I would remain childless. I even learned to enjoy the fact that we did not have children. We were much closer than most couples who did. We were best friends.

We were together all the time and truly enjoyed each other's companionship. That was why his death was so hard. Not only was he a great man, but he was a very good husband and a wonderful friend. He was my entire family.

How could God take away my life like that? Sure, we had our ups and downs, just like every couple. But through the years we had developed a deeper love than I ever knew existed. We also respected each other. Our relationship had evolved into something that we both treasured. Sid would often say how lucky we were that we had each other.

The counseling and listening to others once again came into play. I discovered that it was perfectly normal to be angry with God over such a devastating loss. That doesn't have anything to do with faith or your spirituality, either. It is human to be angry when your soul mate has been ripped from your life. God understands. He really does.

I was also angry at the world. I continued to hate the fact that other people were happy. It just wasn't fair. I used to be happy and now I was miserable. *How could the world keep on turning*? Mine had stopped. Nothing about my life was fair. And I despised everybody for a while. I would go into a rage when someone would even hint that I should try to start living again. *Why?* I would snap at anyone—even those who were trying to help me.

I discovered, though, that the anger stage was the most cleansing of all the stages of grief. Shock, depression, confusion, and guilt don't make you feel better. Anger does. Or at least, it did for me. The screaming, crying and blaming everybody for what happened seemed to help me. The rage and anger I felt moved me from guilt and depression to the next phase of my awful journey—confusion.

10

Widow Brain

I read somewhere that the confusion stage is often called widow brain. You can't think straight. Simple tasks turn into huge ordeals. You can't remember anything.

You can't concentrate or focus on the task at hand, either. I remember a widow friend of mine telling me it took her four days to get through eighty-four pages of a book. She could not comprehend what she read. Another friend put the orange juice in the pantry, only to discover it three days later.

I tried to fight this stage by staying unbelievably busy. But that just made things worse. The hectic schedule I created for myself helped with the loneliness and depression but it led to even more confusion.

In this stage, I learned again to ask for even more help. The paperwork that follows a death is overwhelming…dealing with the attorney, the accountant, the insurance company, etc. etc. The list was endless. I found that most people were not only willing to help me, they wanted to. They just needed to feel like they were doing something—anything--to make this situation better for me.

Sid had his own business and handling that was probably the most difficult and confusing task I had to complete. He had tried over and over again to get me to be more involved with his books, but I never had time. Now it was coming back to bite me. But with the help of his partner, a good accountant, and the attorney, we got Sid's part of the business shut down. When that happened, I felt tremendous relief.

It was quite painful, though, as we sifted through the papers with his signature on them. I think what got to me the most was when I discovered a notepad covered with his famous little circle doodles. So Sid. So sad.

I leaned on other people to help me through the maze of confusion. My brother helped me deal with Social Security and the life insurance company. A friend helped me understand car issues, like when to get my oil changed. I had to learn some things for the first time at the age of fifty-seven.

Sid's best friend since childhood helped me with the many financial hurdles I had to jump over. He even taught me how to create a budget, read our IRA statements and deal with a financial advisor. Those financial issues were the worst to me. The life insurance money was helpful, but my monthly income had been reduced tremendously. I had to face some decisions about money that I detested and feared. But it was up to me. I had to learn to take care of myself.

It took a lot of tears, frustration and time, but I learned how to do all the things that Sid had always done. I discovered that, with help, I could take over his responsibilities.

During the confusion stage, I also

struggled with questions about the future. *Why I am still here? What am I going to do with the rest of my life? What purpose do I have now*? *Will I ever be happy again?*

One day I was driving to work and talking to Sid. I often talked to Sid. It just made me feel better. I began to tear up and I think I said something aloud like, “How can I ever be happy again without you? I can’t imagine that will be possible. Will it?”

About that time, a car passed me. The first part of the license plate read “SJB.” I lost my breath. My heart began racing and I almost choked. Those were Sid’s initials. The name of his company was SJB. *Sid, are you there? You are, aren’t you?*

Some people would say that was just a coincidence. Maybe it was. But I don’t care. I believe it was Sid reaching out to me, telling me that he was okay and that I was going to be okay, too.

It wasn’t like a movie with a happily ever after ending or anything like that. There would still be some very rough days ahead. But it was a turning point for me. It gave me comfort. I began to believe that I was actually somehow, some way, going to make it through this awful gut-wrenching thing called grief.

11

The Gun, the Cigarette Butt, and the Doctor

Other strange things happened to me after the incident with the license plate. Even though I had never really believed such things before, I felt like Sid kept trying to connect with me. When I hesitantly shared some of my experiences with members of my support group, I was surprised to find out that almost everyone had similar stories to tell.

One widow kept hearing a particular old song on the radio—the one she and her husband had picked as their song years earlier. Another member of the group would wake up in the night and smell her dead husband's cigarette smoke. We all agreed that no matter what anyone said, we were comforted by these occurrences.

One thing that happened to me involved friends we had known since college forty years earlier. Jim and Loretta wanted to get married when they were freshmen but didn't have the money for the license, so Sid bought a shotgun from Jim for ten dollars. Shortly after Sid died, Jim and Loretta came to visit me. One morning, Jim came out of the guest room with tears in his eyes, whispering "My gun is in that closet. The one I sold to Sid years ago so I could marry Loretta."

I didn't even realize Sid still had that gun and certainly didn't know it was in that closet. Jim said it was as if things had come full circle and that Sid had made sure he would find the gun. I gave it back to Jim, and he said it was the most wonderful gift he had ever received. He felt like Sid was reaching out to him, too. Sid was still with us, and the gun turning up in the guest room closet was not a coincidence—at least not to me, Jim or Loretta.

Finding one of Sid's cigarette butts was even more bizarre. Sid smoked a certain brand and I would get so irritated when I would find those butts in the driveway. So, he began making sure the butts were put in the trash can in our garage.

It had been months since Sid had died, and no one had smoked anywhere near our house since his death. One morning when I was emptying the garage trash can, I pulled out the liner I had just put there earlier in the week. I was startled to see that distinctive cigarette butt in the bottom of the can.

How could that have just appeared? I emptied that can every week. Sid's cigarette butt had not been there the week before or any other previous week. *Was he speaking to me again?* Just like with the license plate, I was convinced that he was.

But the most amazing experience I had was with a woman named Sandy. I had been introduced to her by my neighbor Marsha. We enjoyed going out to eat, and one night

Sandy mentioned that her son was an emergency room doctor at our local hospital. It didn't hit me until later that Sandy's last name was the same as the doctor who tried to revive Sid that awful November morning.

When I finally put two and two together, I could not bring myself to tell Sandy in person that I knew she was the mother of the doctor who said the words that would change my life forever, "I'm sorry. We did everything we could…."

Sandy's son had been very kind and had tried to comfort me, despite the cold surroundings and proceedings that are necessary after someone has been pronounced dead in a hospital. I actually remember how he gently took my hand and told me, "Don't go there," when I began screaming that it was my fault Sid died.

One day I got my courage up and called Sandy, desperately trying not to let her hear my voice crack with emotion. But we both ended up crying about the fact that we had become friends without even knowing about our other sad connection.

As odd as it might sound, these strange

and eerie events gave me great peace in the midst of all the confusion that followed the loss of my Sid. And that was all that mattered to me.

12

Skin Hunger, Sex, and Safeguarding

The confusion stage, for me, went a lot deeper than just forgetting where I put those important papers or why I came to the store in the first place. It also involved some very complex issues that I was totally unprepared to deal with.

Luckily, again, through literature, counseling, other widows and my grief group, I learned that my desire to be touched was totally normal. It was called skin hunger and many people experienced this during their grief.

We all crave the human touch and without it we feel like we are not loved or needed. It is just a basic human thing. I discovered that this need for touch was particularly important when your partner had been physically affectionate. Sid had always been just that.

I would pass by him and he would grab my hand and kiss it. He would stroke my arm. Sid often touched my face and told me how beautiful I looked. He was emotionally and physically nurturing.

I found myself longing for a hug—particularly from a man. It wasn't anything unusual on my part. I needed that human contact and connection that I was no longer getting.

One of the things that helped me with this issue was the fact that everyone else who had experienced the same kind of loss felt the same way. So, hugs became a huge part of our weekly dinner meetings with my group. And when I met other widows for lunch, we all instinctively embraced each other.

The safeguarding came into play for me

when I tried to protect myself from certain feelings. It hurt so much to remember our good times. So for a while I spent most of my time trying to do anything I could to keep from thinking about Sid and our life together.

That may sound ridiculous, but it just seemed to send me back into that deep dark hole of depression to think about what I had no more. It was unbearable, so I pushed all the hurtful feelings aside. I had wanted to talk about him all the time, and then I didn't. *What the hell did I want, anyway?* All these mixed-up, back-and-forth feelings were totally confusing and frightening.

Another thing that completely took me by surprise was how much I missed having sex. I was raised to believe that was such a personal subject that it should never be discussed with anyone. For the most part, I think that is true. However, when I started thinking about sex a lot, it horrified me. *What was wrong with me? I was supposed to be grieving! How could I even think about such things? I must be a terrible person.*

My friend, Linda, who had been widowed twelve years earlier, set me straight on the sex issue. She said she went through the same thing. She believed that it was her mind's way of saying, "Hey, wake up! I'm still alive here! I can still feel things other than sadness!"

That helped me to realize that thinking about sex more than I had in years was normal and, for some people, a part of the grieving process.

Linda believed it was actually a sign that you were starting to recover. Expressing a need for a basic human experience, like sex, meant that you were slowly heading toward some kind of life again. The danger in it, of course, was making sure you didn't act on those sexual feelings until you were ready. Like Linda said, when you are in that grieving process your emotions are upside down, and you need to wait until they are right side up before you enter any kind of relationship.

Thank you, Linda. You made me breathe a sigh of relief and see that I wasn't nuts or twisted after all.

13

God Has a Sense of Humor and "By the Way, I know a Nice Guy..."

In all the confusion, I began to experience lighter times more often. It felt good to laugh once in a while. The bad days were still there, of course, and always would be, just like the minefield. But I could actually have a really good day here and there.

One of the things that seemed to keep me going as I slowly progressed down my "grief road" was the fact that I think God began doing things to entertain me. At almost fifty-eight, I certainly did not think of myself as that desirable. Of course, I was to Sid. But he saw past the wrinkles and the extra weight. He loved me for what I was inside, not outside.

So it surprised me when men started to come out of the woodwork. It wasn't just me. Many other widows I knew were experiencing the same thing. Men were approaching them, and their friends were trying to fix them up with "nice guys" they knew.

We widows would often get together and compare notes about the bombardment of men after you lose your husband. Was it because they thought we were helpless without them?

Were they after the money they imagined you had? Did they just think we were lonely? Or was it something else….

One friend met me for lunch and pulled up her bangs, asking, "Do you see 'widow desperate for sex' tattooed across my forehead?" I laughed so hard as she explained that at almost seventy, she was being propositioned right and left by the opposite sex. We all had to admit that it w a great diversion. God had a sense of humor. He thought we needed some laughter in our lives. So it began raining men who came armed with classic pick-up lines!

I heard from old high school boyfriends I hadn't seen in forty years. Men that I thought were friends of Sid's suddenly wanted to "be more." I was a "fox," a "babe" and "drop-dead gorgeous" at almost sixty! Some things never change, including the lines and the games. This entertaining nonsense came into my life at the right time. I was ready for some fun.

Everyone from my hairdresser and coworkers, to neighbors and friends knew a great guy that would just be perfect for me. I heard things like: "Oh—well, yes he did spend one night in jail, but it wasn't his fault," and, "He has three grown unemployed kids who all live with him, but that is just because he has a big heart. Trust me!" Even one of the male members of our grief group had a guy from church he wanted to introduce me to, until he discovered the guy was a lot younger than he looked and I was old enough to be his mother!

When these "fix-up" attempts would take place, I would just politely smile and say "Thank you, but I'm not ready." And that was the truth. But all the male attention was fun, and it did make me think about the future as I had never thought about it before during this journey. Sid was the love of my life. *How could I ever love anyone again? Would that be possible? Wouldn't I be constantly comparing someone new to my wonderful Sid? Would I even want another man in my life now that I knew I could actually take care of myself?*

I didn't know the answers and wouldn't for a very long time. But at least I was thinking about the future. That was important. I thought my life had stopped the day Sid died. But I slowly came to the realization that life would go on for me. I just had to be patient, have faith, figure out how I wanted to spend the rest of my life, and proceed from there.

14

Family and Friends

When you suffer such a devastating loss, the support of family and friends is, to me, the only way you end up surviving at all.

You expect your family to be there for you, but what my family did for me was so amazing. They came as quickly as they could from all over the United States. My sister Laura was getting ready to go to the airport to fly to my mother's home in Idaho for Thanksgiving when she got the news about Sid's death. How she managed to get a last minute ticket during the holidays to come to my side I don't know. And I hate to think about what it cost her and my brother, too. Laura spent the next several days helping me emotionally and physically, working constantly to do whatever I needed her to do.

My brother, Sean, was my rock. Nine years my junior, he became my "big brother" right after Sid died. He came immediately, too, coordinated everything, and officiated at the memorial service. And later, he was always there when I had a problem or question that I thought needed a man's opinion.

Our friends Steve and Kathy drove up from Alabama and stayed by my side for days. Another friend, David, came from Florida and did the same thing. Sid and I had plans to spend Thanksgiving that year with Jeff and Becki. I couldn't believe it when Becki, who had also spent hours helping my sister, called and said we were still having Thanksgiving dinner together. They arrived with a vanload of food and even brought tables and chairs from Jeff's office. They generously provided dinner for my family and the out-of-town company we had.

I could not believe how many people

came to Sid's memorial service the day after Thanksgiving—former employees of his, my co-workers, friends, neighbors, friends of friends and the list goes on and on. They gave up their family time to be with me and support me. Each face I saw, each hug I got enveloped me with love.

So many people spoke at Sid's memorial —his business partner, George; our friend, Jeff; my sister-in-law Becky and her son, Grant. Becky's father had died just days earlier, and she had left her home in North Carolina to attend his funeral in Texas. As soon as her father's funeral was over, Becky flew directly to Tennessee to be at Sid's service. All four of my nephews, including Grant, drove from North Carolina to be there for me.

And Steve, a dear friend from college, gave the most wonderful eulogy. It was funny, sweet, loving, and so perfect for Sid. Another friend, also named Steve, provided a beautiful musical tribute at the memorial.

My mother, who had just lost my father six weeks earlier, came from Idaho. She was worn out, as dad had suffered from

Alzheimer's for years. Yet, she came to Tennessee to be with me for the memorial service and then flew with me to Texas for the graveside service.

My ex-sister-in-law, Eddie, who had been my best friend since we were eighteen, met us at the airport and took care of us in Texas. Her concern and support for me never stopped. We may not have been officially related anymore, but she continued to call me, check on me and constantly encourage me like a sister. She still does.

My sister Charisse and my niece, Simone, drove for hours to be at the graveside service, and Charisse gave such a touching speech about Sid's deep love for me. Sid's cousins John and Mari Lyn were there, and John preached a lovely sermon that was just exactly what Sid would have wanted.

Many friends and family members had traveled hundreds of miles to be at the graveside service, and some were elderly and not in the best of health. But they came to honor Sid. Even many members of his college football team from forty years earlier were there.

In the months that followed, I had more support than I could ever describe. Without it, healing would not have been possible.

Even my best buddy and confidant from high school, Bill, contacted me from Oregon after he heard about Sid. He and his wife Sharon, became my "unexpected angels." I had not seen Bill in twenty years and had only met her once, yet their comforting calls and e-mails were never ending. I always felt like Sid had a hand in bringing Bill back into my life at a time when I needed him the most.

But my neighbor Marsha and her son Bryson were the ones who became my everyday steady support. What they did for me can never ever be put into words. They were always there for me—always. Sid would be so proud of how they took care of me, loved me like family, and held my hand every step of the way.

Sid was a solitary man, and used to joke around saying he didn't know who would bother to come to his funeral. At one point when my house was completely overrun with people, someone repeated that comment and added: “Look down, Sid!”

He was loved by so many people, and so was I.

15

Playing the Widow Card

The sympathy, understanding and help you get when you become a widow are so important, but these wonderful expressions of support can also lead to leaning on people too much. I would call that "playing the widow card." At first it is not only normal but to be expected. As they told us in our grief support group, "Be selfish for a while. It is okay." And I had learned to do just that and accept help.

I remember how I fell apart at the bank

the first time I had to deal with my statement and order checks with just my name on them. I couldn't even understand the instructions or fill out the order form. So I let the branch manager do those things for me as I sat across from her crying my eyes out.

Physical help, like a neighbor offering to mow the lawn is fine, too, in the early months following such a loss. But after a while, if you play the widow card too much, you can become too dependent on family members and friends to take care of your needs. You don't want your helplessness to become so tiresome that people begin to avoid you.

It is so easy to wallow in your grief and let everyone else take over. To me, starting to live by myself was like trying to learn how to ride a bike. At some point, you have to tell the person pushing the bike for you to let go. I had to start hanging on to that wobbly bike and ride it all by myself if I were to achieve independence. Months went by and it was time for me to try to stand on my own a little. It was a tedious process, too. As one widowed friend put it, "Just take baby steps."

So I did. And at first, I fell off that bike a lot. But I tried to get right back on it. A neighbor showed me how to use the weed-eater, and I tried to resist making those late night phone calls just because I was desperately lonely.

From other widows, I learned some things I shouldn't do. I met one woman who had been widowed years earlier. Yet she seemed still stuck in that anger and helpless depression rut. Another widow told me, "Getting better starts with you. You have to have a positive attitude, be willing to learn new things, be proud of your accomplishments, and try to remember that Sid would want you to keep going."

I quickly figured out that aligning myself with negative people was counter-productive for me in the healing process. I began to try to surround myself with positive people who would keep me feeling up. I could not afford to be dragged down—not even by another widow. We could help each other, but if only one of us was willing to try, it wasn't going to work for either of us.

A friend who had been widowed twenty years earlier called me one day. Dot said that one of the ways she played the widow card was deciding that when her husband died, he immediately became a saint. That was something Sid had said he did not want me to do. Of course Dot did not do this consciously, but came to the realization that she had built her husband up to be some sort of super human being that could do no wrong. It caused her to be unhappy with everyone. No one in her life could measure up to her husband, and when she started to date, it became a real issue.

Dot said when she became aware of the problem; she embraced the fact that her husband had not been perfect. Remember his faults. Laugh about the quirky things he did. And if you do decide to date, enjoy the differences—don't compare them. If you do that, the dead saintly husband will win every time, and you might miss out on something wonderful that is right in front of you.

Playing the widow card, however, could be a real advantage at times, and I must admit I used it. I remember when I was dealing with the phone company and trying to get Sid's business line disconnected. It was heart wrenching to do that—another awful task that had to be tackled and one more of those damn mines I had to step on. The representative took care of my request, but then proceeded to try to sell me their computer connection service. "Excuse me!" I shouted. "My husband just died and you are trying to sell me something? What kind of a person are you?" Needless to say, the sales pitch came to an immediate halt.

Playing the widow card did have its place.

16

Here's What I Think You Should Do

Another problem with playing the widow card too much and too long is that you open yourself up to a lot of unwanted advice. Of course unsolicited advice actually starts early on, as one friend discovered when the non-traditional funeral she planned for her husband did not meet with the approval of some conservative friends and family members.

As time went on, I was bombarded with everything from "You should move" and

"You should consider dating again right away" to "Just take a cruise and forget everything for a while" and "You need to get a dog."

One widow said she felt like the only words she heard for a while were "you should" or "you shouldn't," and it made her confusion even worse. In your grief, sometimes it is hard to stand up for yourself, but at some point, you have just say "Thank you," and then do what you think is best for you.

From spiritual needs to financial plans, each widow must stop and breathe as my friend Elizabeth so wisely told me, and approach each day individually. It is hard enough to make it through the maze of grief as it is, without allowing someone to control your direction and decisions. When I reached a place where I had conquered widow brain and put away my widow card, I took the time to rewind so I could move forward. I reflected on what had happened and what needed to happen. I stopped and I breathed.

Loving Sid had completed me. I did not feel whole without him. *What did I need to do to be able to move on? How could I face the future and what future would there be without Sid?* Advice was great, but in the end I had to figure these things out for myself. So I learned to take it all in, sift through comments about what I should or shouldn't do and come up with my own plan for the rest of my life. As they had told us in the grief group, we all shared a common bond, yet each one of us would have to find our own path to healing. What worked for one person might not work for another.

I decided, though, some of the dos and don'ts were valid. For example, don't let strangers know you live alone. Ask friends for the names of people they trust to do things like repair work. And when a person gives you a quote on something, don't be afraid to say, "Let me ask my husband." It isn't just the danger aspect, but also the fact that sometimes people have a tendency to take advantage of widows. It doesn't hurt to ask friends if a quoted price is actually fair.

Another piece of advice I found important was don't tell anyone how much money you have. First, it isn't anyone's business, and second, it could also lead to someone taking advantage of your situation. Understand exactly what you have and don't turn over control of all your money to anyone was another comment I took to heart. This does not mean a trusted family member or reputable financial advisor cannot be helpful, but you have to know what your assets and debts are, what you need to live on and what you want to happen with your money. You have to stay in control and speak up concerning financial decisions.

An important "should do" was educate yourself. Learn all you can about financial issues that will help your situation. Another great piece of advice I was given was not to make any major financial decisions for a while, and I didn't.

Dating was another thing that I found to be unique to each widow. I knew two who married less than a year after losing their husbands. Another woman who had been widowed for almost fifteen years was very happy with her single life and did not date at all.

Some of my widowed friends found

taking anti-depressants was very helpful for them. Others believed that those types of medications were not what they needed during the grief process. Even smaller issues are individual. One widow I knew cleaned out her husband's closet the day after the funeral. For me, it took almost a year. No one can tell you when it is the right time to do anything.

I listened, learned, trusted my instincts, and then made my own decisions. That led me a few steps down the road to another place where I felt a little more confident and contented.

17

They Call it Happiness Guilt

Just about the time I started to feel like living again, I ran into what they call happiness guilt. Thank goodness the counselors had warned us about that. It was just another turn on the road to recovery. I had dragged myself through the shock, depression, guilt, anger and confusion only to reach this roadblock. I was finally making some progress building a new life for myself, and then it hit me.

Sid worked out of our home, and I only worked at our local library eight hours a week. We were rarely apart and ate most of our meals together. And because we didn't have children, we spent a lot of time sharing things we enjoyed like flea markets, auctions, and festivals. We were closer than any couple I knew. But that closeness made the loneliness so much deeper. It was also hard because most of my family lived halfway across the country.

I found myself doing anything to stay out of the big empty house that had once been filled by Sid's deep booming laugh. I used to joke with him, telling him that I needed some "alone time." Be careful what you wish for. I ended up with all the alone time in the world and I hated it. I was not used to being alone. I lived for the days I worked and despised the days I didn't. Weekends were absolute hell.

Of course it helped tremendously to have Marsha and Bryson across the street. They were always including me in their activities and taking me to dinner, or out shopping. They were constant companions. And other people continued to contact me regularly. I looked forward to e-mails and hearing cheery voices on the phone. As well as my family members, more than a dozen friends stayed in touch with me. My friend Loretta even came from Texas a few months after Sid died just to offer me her love and support.

I began to develop new friendships with other widows. We had a sad bond, but sometimes it was easier to be around people who understood so well what I was going through. But it wasn't enough. I missed my friend, my lover, my soul mate. Many days I still couldn't imagine how I would ever manage without Sid. I would often catch myself thinking things like *this time last year we were enjoying those great corndogs at the state fair and we were happy*.

Almost nine months after Sid died I spent an entire day alone, something that I had been avoiding. I had a few phone conversations, but that was all. It suddenly hit me. I was alone and I wasn't totally unhappy. I felt so guilty. *Did this mean I didn't miss him enough? Why wasn't I miserable today as I had been every other day I had spent alone? This can't be right!* But it was, and I realized I was suffering from my first taste of happiness guilt. I was okay being alone. Definitely not giddy and joyful—but fairly contented. And I felt horrible about it.

But I remembered what my grief counselor, Pam, had said about happiness guilt. I knew that it didn't mean that I didn't miss Sid. I did. It was just that my new normal life was continuing to evolve and I was learning how to cope with my loss. She had also explained to our group that we had to think about how we would feel if we had been the ones to die. Would we want our loved ones to be unhappy and never move on? Of course not.

No one ever gets over a death. But I learned that we have to find a way to go on and be happy again. We have no choice. The alternative is to be miserable until we die. If we live out our remaining days bitterly unhappy, we were virtually dead, too. I had to live again.

There would be a lot more happiness guilt ahead. I knew I had accepted that when I responded to the questionnaire sent by my fortieth high school reunion committee with the words: "I hope to honor my husband's memory by making the most out of the rest of my life."

18

Taking and Giving Emotional Support

So many widows came forward to help me when I became one. My friend Elizabeth was always telling me that I would be all right and helping me understand that, although we shared the same journey, our paths would be different. And that was okay too. She led me to some websites especially for young widows, and many friends sent helpful books and articles. I read them all.

My sister-in-law, Becky, had lost Sid's brother less than four years earlier. Right after Sid died; she held me tightly and whispered, "It will be better." It is easier to see there is hope when it comes from someone who has walked in your shoes.

My friend Kathie validated my feelings by telling me that she, too, had felt like her life was over and that she was old, ugly and no one would ever want or love her again. She did find love again, and even if that wasn't meant to be for me, it made me realize that it was actually possible.

Even my accountant reached out to me. She had lost her husband ten years earlier and understood my confusion and helplessness in dealing with issues like finances and taxes. She made me believe I could handle all those things, and eventually I did.

It was particularly helpful to hear from those younger widows. They understood the uniqueness of becoming a widow years before you thought you would. Not that being widowed at any time was okay. It was just that there were different issues to deal with when your spouse died thirty years before he was supposed to.

One of the worst things about losing Sid was that suddenly no one needed me. I felt like the one and only person who really depended on me was gone, and so was my main purpose in life.

One day Pam called me and asked if she could refer Nancy, a newly widowed woman who was also in her fifties, to me. Nancy was having a rough time, and Pam thought I could help her.

Somebody needed me! It was so wonderful, and Nancy and I immediately connected. I was four months farther down the road on this journey. I could tell her things that hopefully would allow her to see that there truly was light at the end of the awful, deep, dark tunnel called grief.

About the same time, I found out a very close friend from high school, Rich, had died in New York. I had not seen Rich in forty years, but he had always been there for me in high school. I had thought about him so much over the years. I contacted his widow, Pat, and we began to correspond. We had never met, yet she came down for a visit. She said she felt this overwhelming need to be with someone who understood her pain. We talked and cried and shared. Pat and I decided that Sid and Rich were probably up there "high fiving" it and proud of themselves for putting us together. And when she left I felt like I had not just helped her by offering advice and support. Hopefully, I had also returned the kindness of friendship that her husband had given to me so long ago. Something good had come out of two very bad losses.

It felt wonderful to finally begin to truly get out of the "all-about-me" mode. When you have suffered through such a traumatic experience, it is so easy to stay in a place where you can't stop feeling sorry for yourself. It was time for me to realize that other people had problems, too, and I had to try to help. By helping others, I helped myself. I felt needed. I saw how far I had come in the process, too, and discovered that there is nothing more healing than helping other people.

19

I Can Live Without You - I Just Don't Want To

When I heard the line, "I can live without you. I just don't want to," in a movie, I thought it spoke to me. I had reached a point where I knew I could handle myself and all our business. I had gained so much confidence since Sid died. I had seen a chart called the grief circle that expressed the many stages of grief that would eventually lead you back to some kind of life. The last phase involved personal growth and reconciliation.

I believed I had grown as a person and the reconciliation was beginning to take hold, too. I no longer had nearly as much sadness, anger, and guilt. Instead, I began to treasure the thirty-eight years I had with the man who adored me. *How many people can say they had that?*

I remembered a passage I had read in Tim Russert's book *Big Russ and Me* about a friend who had lost a child. He was asked to consider whether he would have made a deal with God when that child was born. If God had told him up front that he would give him this precious child to love—only to take him away too early, would he still want the child?

The answer, of course, was yes. That made an impact on me. I started thinking about all the years I had with Sid and how wonderful they were, instead of all the years that we would never have together. *How lucky I was to have those years.*

The thoughts I had tried so hard to suppress months earlier became comforting to me. I would smile, recalling the many good times we shared. Memories became warm and comforting instead of terribly painful. They still hurt, but I had come so far. There would always be a scar from that awful, deep wound. But I was healing more and more each day from losing the person I loved more than anyone else in the world.

Some important words on the grief cycle were "renew and reorganize." I was starting to feel renewed and reorganized. I began to do the things I once loved again, like my genealogy and writing. I was thinking about what would make me happy and how I could achieve that. I even considered new things I could try. When my friend, Sandy, suggested we take line dancing lessons together, I thought, *Why not?* It would be fun to try something I had never tried before. It was invigorating to think about new possibilities in my life, even if they were small.

There was life after death. I could finally see that. But still, it wasn't the life I wanted. I knew in my heart that if I could go back, I would in an instant. Things had been so right before. I was doing okay and moving ahead, but I did not like my new life as much as I had the old one.

I realized that I wasn't quite where I

wanted to be. I looked at the chart and saw the last part of the cycle, "acceptance and rebirth." I hadn't totally accepted Sid's death and although I was feeling renewed, I wasn't feeling reborn yet. But that was all right. I had come such a long way and been through so much. I knew Sid would be proud of me.

It helped when I heard the words of another person who had traveled the same road. My sister Laura was telling a widowed co-worker about my loss, and she said, "Tell your sister it won't ever be the same. But she will learn that life can be good again and she can be happy in a different way."

I couldn't turn back time. My journey would never really be over, but I had to find a way to make it to that final place on the grief cycle, the one that was marked "acceptance and rebirth." I owed it to my husband, Sid. *He was counting on me to make it all the way through this.*

20

Acceptance and Rebirth

I read in one grief book that when a widow does something with her wedding ring, she has accepted the death of her husband. I don't think that is necessarily true. But the wedding ring issue is one that most widows I met brought up at one time or another.

Do I keep it on my left hand? Do I have it restyled? Do I put it away and never wear it at all? I came to understand that each widow deals with her wedding ring differently, and there is no time schedule concerning this aspect of losing your husband. One woman I knew was still wearing her wedding ring on her left hand five years after the death of her husband. Another immediately had hers made into a dinner ring that she wore on her left hand. One friend added gemstones to the setting and wore that new ring on her right hand.

It wasn't a conscious decision on my part, but one day about six months after Sid died I just moved my wedding ring to my right hand. I don't know why or what made me do that. I know that it did not mean that I had accepted his death completely. I had not. Maybe it just meant that I was getting closer to really believing he was gone, and moving my ring at that particular time just felt right. I decided not to question it.

Early on, my grief counselor Pam told me that one day I would probably feel reborn—just like the chart said. At the time, I thought she had lost her mind. *Reborn? What the hell was she talking about? I liked my life with Sid just the way it was, thank you.*

As the months went by I began to understand that acceptance needs to happen, as it is the vehicle that slowly leads you to rebirth. Plan A for your life fades from your memory and plan B emerges and takes over.

You don't just wake up one day and announce, "I have accepted this, and I am reborn!" For me it was a long, unpredictable process that sometimes seemed liked one step forward and two steps back. I would feel so confident and self-assured one day and then I would slip into the "I can't do this" mode the next. It also does not mean that you wipe out your old life. Of course you don't, but you learn that your heart is big enough to hold those precious memories of your husband as well as hope and happiness for your new life without him.

Sid had always been my biggest fan. He gave me confidence and supported everything I did. We had been together since we were teenagers, and I felt so lost at first without the person who kept up my self-esteem and made me feel like I could do anything. Wise words from Pam helped me. She told me to learn to love myself as much as Sid loved me. It wasn't easy but I began to see that I was my own person, and the qualities that Sid loved in me were still there. I also realized that I had developed new abilities.

Sid's death had devastated, but not defeated, me. I had stumbled many times, but with a lot of help, I had gotten up and kept going. I was stronger. I was wiser. I was smarter, and I was surer of myself.

For a while, close friends and family members worried constantly and tried to protect me from the real world. One person said, "I just don't want you to get your heart broken over anything." But when your heart has been totally shattered like mine was, it can never really be broken again. Your worst fear has been realized, and somehow, that makes you stronger, too.

Close to a year after he died, I finally accepted that Sid would never come back to me in this life. I could hear the word "widow" and not break down uncontrollably like I had done the first time I was called that by a probate judge. At a family wedding, it suddenly dawned on me that if I wanted to, I could stand behind the bride with the other single women when she tossed her bouquet.

My friend Diana and I had written a song about loss several years earlier that we played at Sid's memorial, because he loved it so much. The song ended up being sadly prophetic.

"Just a Smile Away" was the title, and the words in the chorus became my theme of acceptance: "And when I need to see you, I won't have to look too far. You're right here in my heart—just a smile away."

Sid was truly, physically, completely gone. Yet I was comforted by the fact that he would never really leave me. I had embraced acceptance and that would lead me to the final word on the grief cycle chart—rebirth. But it would take stepping back in time for me to move forward and reach that last stage.

21

A Time to be Reborn

I never dreamed I would go to my fortieth class reunion as a widow. When I first got the notice from my high school in Eugene, Oregon, Sid had been gone only a few months. I could not imagine traveling all the way from Tennessee to face people I had not seen in decades and trying to handle very painful questions like, “Are you married?”

When the time came for the reunion, I was much farther along in my journey. Many classmates had also contacted me, offering their sympathy and understanding. Sid grew up in Texas, and most of my high school friends had never met him. I had attended high school in Oregon only two years, so I was very grateful that people from my distant past had reached out to me. I was eager to see classmates I had kept in close contact with, like my best friend Kathie. She was coming all the way from Hawaii, and we planned to attend the festivities together. And then there was my dear friend Bill, who had re-entered my life and been such a support in the months following Sid's death.

It turned out to be perfect timing for me to attend the class reunion. I was finally ready to step out and have some real fun, and I wanted to thank those special classmates for their support and encouragement. For the first time, I felt like I could really stand on my own. My friend Diana said she thought it was interesting that "reborn" and "reunion" both began with the same prefix. I had never thought of those two things together. But I began to see that the reunion was my chance to feel reborn again.

I could not face eating alone after Sid died and I had lost fifteen pounds. I bought some clothes that were much more stylish and "hot" and got a new hairstyle. I took my friend Sharon's advice and began starting each day by standing in front of the mirror and declaring, "I am woman—hear me roar!"

Maybe I was pushing sixty, but I was determined to look as vibrant, smart, and confident as possible. The journey had been difficult and still was at times. But I had truly grown into a different person and wanted the self-assurance I felt on the inside to show on the outside. So I threw my shoulders back and forged ahead. *South Eugene High School Class of 1966, here I come! Get ready*!

I had not seen my friends Kathie and Bill in twenty years, yet time melted away the instant I saw them at the airport. We were so bonded from supporting each other during those turbulent teenage years. We joyfully embraced and picked up right where we left off.

Visiting with them was easy and I was equally relaxed getting together with other friends. We laughed about old times and shared photos of our families, and they comforted me.

Several events were being held simultaneously on the first official night of the reunion. I had chosen to attend the pub gathering and when I realized I would be walking into that alone, I began to panic. Even though I was more outgoing than Sid, he had always been there at my side in social situations. *How could I do this without him?* This time I would not be on his arm where I could turn and look at his approving smile.

My hands were shaking so hard as I drove the rental car to the pub that I could hardly hold on to the steering wheel. Then I remembered Elizabeth's advice—*stop and breathe*. And Kathie, sweet wonderful Kathie, who was always there for me, had once again boosted my confidence by giving me a pep talk back at the motel, "You can do this," she said. "You truly are stronger and wiser now, so don't be afraid." I parked the car and said a little prayer.

It wasn't as if everything fell right into place the minute I walked in and saw my classmates. My knees were shaking and my palms were moist. But as I began to recognize people from my past, excitement overcame the fear. There were squeals, hugs, and questions about jobs, kids, and grandkids. We shared “Remember when?” and “Can you believe we did that?” I heard a strong confident voice and then I realized it was my voice. My new voice. The new normal.

There I was all alone. I was interacting with people and handling myself intelligently. I even managed to answer questions about Sid with dignity and grace. I discovered that I could be witty and charming, too. It was so wonderfully empowering.

Late in the evening I excused myself and went to the powder room. I stopped abruptly when I saw a reflection in the mirror. *Who was that woman?* It wasn’t the cowering teenager with self-esteem issues who married her knight in shining armor. Staring back at me was a real grown-up woman who stood straight and tall. *God, I don’t even recognize myself.* It was a strange, yet great, feeling.

I knew there would always be times when deep sadness would overtake me. But I also realized that moment was another turning point on the road to a new happy life. I had suffered devastating injuries crossing the worst part of the minefield. I had nursed those wounds and I wasn't as good as new—I was better.

22

The New Me

The first year after Sid died dragged on. I felt like each day was a week long. But time continued to be a great healer. My life slowly got even better. I also started to discover more about the new me-- the one who began emerging at my reunion. And, as sad as it was, this new woman had accepted the fact that she was no longer Sid's wife. She was his widow and had to keep rebuilding her life.

The stronger I became the more new challenges I had to face. And I had to make some tough decisions that were painful. I sold the home Sid and I had shared in Tennessee for almost twelve years, moved to Texas, and bought a new house that was much more suitable for a single woman. I found new friends, took up new interests and began dating. It wasn't that simple or easy, but for me personally, these changes helped me as I struggled to pick myself up from the far side of the minefield.

Like other milestones on the journey through grief, these decisions are very personal. Some widows find it helpful to stay in the home they owned with their husbands. Others, like me, want a fresh start after such a loss. Some find comfort and are able to begin again in familiar surroundings. I needed a totally new place. I knew that also meant I would step on another mine, and this time I would be putting that mine right in front of me. But I had to walk through this explosion of grief to really move on with my life.

My friend Loretta flew to Tennessee from Texas and was with me the day the movers packed up my house. It was so sad to say goodbye to my friends and our home.

When I hugged my neighbors Marsha and Bryson, I cried harder than I had since the day Sid died. Loretta helped me so much and even drove all the way back to my new home in Tyler, Texas with me. As she helped me on this part of my journey, I could not imagine that I would soon suffer another devastating loss.

Loretta had been seriously ill for some time but had been in remission for a while. We were all praying that it would last. Sadly, it did not. Just a few weeks after she and I returned to Texas, she was back at M.D. Anderson Hospital in Houston where she remained until two weeks before her death. I saw her several times in those last few months. The last time was at her home a week before she died. There were so many things I wanted her to know, like how much I appreciated her help and support during such a difficult time. But most of all, I wanted her to know that I loved her. And she told me how proud she was of the new person I had become. At least with Loretta, I had the chance to say goodbye.

Loretta died on Father's Day. Her

husband, Jim, told me that when Loretta was dying, she reached up with her arms like someone was beckoning her. Jim believed it was Sid telling her, "Come on my friend. It is okay and I will be here to help you." It gave us both such comfort.

With the exception of Loretta's death, the second year was much easier for me than the first. I knew that no matter how much time passed, occasionally I would step on a mine like I did when I moved and Loretta died, but that was normal.

The journey through grief never really ends. Instead it becomes more like a long road you can look back on, rather than a minefield you are struggling to crawl across —even though the road still hides a mine here and there.

The woman who wrote these last chapters has traveled a long way since one horrible moment thrust her onto the minefield of loss. But life is about accepting changes—even the bad ones-- and moving forward with them.

People often told me that there was a reason Sid died. I don't know if I will ever be able to accept the fact that there was a reason I lost my soul mate, lover, and friend. I prefer to think about it in a different way. I believe, instead, that a lot of good came out of something very bad. Sid's death made me discover my strength and confidence. I learned to love myself as much as Sid loved me, as my grief counselor, Pam, had advised me to do. And I continued to find that my experience in crossing the minefield could help others who had suffered such a loss. Only a person who has walked down the same path truly understands.

Almost two years after Sid died I went to the cemetery with a man. Someone I cared about very much. I was finally happy again, but the visit to Sid's grave triggered another explosion of confusing emotions. *This is so strange. How could I be sitting here sobbing over my husband while in the arms of another man? Is something wrong with me? No, I am just so very blessed to have a beautiful past and a future full of love, hope, and promise.*

I looked up at a stately tree that stood silhouetted against a beautiful blue sky. *Just like my Sid. Proud and confident.* I felt my tears roll down across what I realized was a smile. Sid would always be with me because he left me such wonderful memories. *Just a smile away.*

And I knew Sid would be proud of me, too. The happiness guilt seemed to float away like the golden leaf that gently fluttered by me. I felt a peaceful, warm breeze kiss my cheek. *He is happy that I am happy.* I knew right down to my very soul that it was my sweet loving Sid saying goodbye and cheering for the new me. *Goodbye baby.*

23

Aftermath

Gone but not forgotten. That is so true. After my journey through the minefield of grief there was aftermath. There always will be.

As the years go by, I look back and see that at times I was a bit naïve about where I was on this path. But I prefer to think, that as unrealistic as it might have been, I was going forward with hope. I just wanted to be happy again and perhaps trying too hard those first few years was better than not trying at all.

Aftermath is described in my well worn dictionary as "a period of time following a disastrous event." For me that "period of time" will be until the day I die. Yes, you must learn to live with grief and if you are successful, you are happy once again.

For the most part, you have crossed the minefield and you are stronger for it. You have the scars to prove it. The explosions hit you less often and they are much less painful as time goes on. Still, you can't forget those awful feelings completely.

Around the holiday season will always be hard for me—the anniversary of Sid's death is November 22nd, his birthday is December 14th and our anniversary is January 27th. Thanksgiving and Christmas thrown into that mix make the sadness deeper. Little things can also remind you of the aftermath, even when your life is going along just fine.

I read in an advice column about something called "pennies from heaven." It may seem ridiculous to some people, but since my husband died, the premise works for me. When you find a penny, pick it up, and look at the year. The idea is that a lost loved one is reaching out to you.

I have had the experience several times of finding a penny, only to see a year stamped on it — one that is meaningful and particularly connected to a special person. Just recently I was running some routine errands when suddenly out of the blue, my thoughts turned to Sid. *If he were here today, would he look the same? He would be so proud of our two new great nieces! Would we still be living in the same home?* My heart was heavy with questions and reflections.

I could almost hear his voice and I wondered what he would say about how the world had changed since he left it. *I wish I could hear him laugh just one more time.*

As I opened the door to my car I saw a penny on the ground. I picked it up and I saw the year. *2005.* The year Sid died. I lost my breath—just like I did that day the car passed me with a license plate bearing Sid's initials, or the time I felt his presence at the cemetery.

I clutched the penny tightly and held it for a few moments next to my racing heart. I closed my eyes and my mind embraced his beautiful smile. I smiled back at him. *You are with me now and always will be. Just a smile away.*

Someone else might dismiss those "pennies from heaven" experiences, but for me I believe I am being touched from beyond. As my grief counselor Pam once told me, it doesn't matter what other people think. Go with your own feelings and do what is best for you. There is nothing wrong with believing something that makes you feel better.

Every time I find a penny—particularly one that I feel is connected to my Sid, I feel comforted. It helps me handle the aftermath.

Epilogue

It has taken me five years to find the courage to write these final words. I have changed so much since that awful November morning that altered the course of my life forever. With determination, support, time, faith and hope, each year has gotten better, although there have—and always will be—struggles along the way. Aftermath.

I have lost several more dear friends. Loretta's husband Jim died suddenly just a year after she did. Julie lost her brave battle with cancer at the age of fifty-eight and Jan's long struggle with health issues finally ended on her seventieth birthday.

But I try to focus on the good things that have happened since Sid died. I continue to evolve and have learned so much about myself. I discovered my inner strength and qualities I never knew I had. I am happily remarried and have four stepchildren and eight grandchildren whom I adore. *Life is good.*

In October of 2010, Sid Bailey was inducted into his college hall of fame for his athletic achievements. Family members and friends traveled to Kilgore College to honor him. We proudly shared our tears of joy and remembrance.

I have tried to emphasize on these pages that everyone's journey through the minefield of grief is different. But I hope this book helps someone else suffering through a loss to find the right fork on the road to recovery.

In summary I would say first, grieve, and don't let anyone else tell you how to do that. Then try to help yourself emerge from the darkness into the light of a new life. Time is a great healer, but it is not enough.

No one and nothing can take that person from you. Sid is not forgotten and never will be, but facing the worst mines head on and surviving them enabled me to become a happy, productive person again—one that can better deal with the explosions of grief that still manage to creep into my life occasionally. And that is what recovery is all about.

You must try to cross the minefield for yourself, as well as for the people who love you. And—the best way to honor your lost loved one is to fight for every step on your journey to find a new, happy life. Those times when a mine knocks you off your feet, pick your battered soul up and bravely walk on, armed with hope, sweet memories and love in your heart. You can make it. I know.

Author Biography

Melinda Richarz Lyons earned a B.A. in Journalism from the University of North Texas, and has been a free lance writer for over forty years. Her articles have appeared in many publications, including *Cats Magazine, True West, Nashville Parent, Frontier Times, Kids, Etc., Reminisce, Chicken Soup for the Soul: True Love* and *Cincinnati Family Magazine.*

In 2004, Ms. Lyons was the co-recipient of the Academy of Western Artists Will Rogers Award for Best Song of the Year. She is the author of the several books, including *Murder at the Oaklands Mansion.* Her most recent work appears in *Chicken Soup for the Soul: Grandmothers.*

She lives in Tyler, Texas with her husband Tom and invites you to visit her website: www.melindalyons.com.

37785597R00079

Made in the USA
Charleston, SC
20 January 2015